Low Fodmap Diet

Delicious And Digestive-friendly Recipes For Growing

Older Gracefully

(A Comprehensive Guide To Enjoying A Life Devoid Of

Symptoms)

Gareth Holdsworth

TABLE OF CONTENT

Introduction

FODMAPs are inadequately assimilated carbohydrates and sugar alcohols of short chain length. They form in the large intestine (bowel) during digestion, consuming water and generating carbon dioxide, hydrogen, and methane gas, which causes the intestinal lumen to enlarge. This results in gastrointestinal symptoms, such as discomfort and pain, that are typical of IBS.

Some foods contain FODMAPs naturally or as an additive. They consist of fructose, fructans, lactose, galactans, and polyols (artificial sweeteners).

Some of these foods contain healthy prebiotics, such as fructans, inulin, and galactooligosaccharides (GOS), which promote the growth of beneficial gut flora. Many of them are healthy, but consuming them can induce gastrointestinal symptoms in some individuals.

The low-FODMAP diet, according to JOHN HOPKIN gastroenterologist HAZEL GALON Veloso, M.D., is a very restrictive temporary dietary plan. Always consult your physician before beginning a new diet, but because the low-FODMAP diet eliminates so many foods, no one should follow it for an extended period. Finding out which foods are problematic for you is a fast process.

Food frequently causes digestive symptoms. Interestingly, restricting a specific food can substantially alleviate these symptoms in hypersensitive individuals.

For the clinical management of irritable bowel syndrome (IBS), a diet deficient in fermentable carbohydrates known as FODMAPS is recommended.

The acronym FODMAP refers to fermentable oligo-, di-, mono-, and polyols.

These are the terms used to classify carbohydrate groups notorious for causing digestive symptoms such as gas, bloating, and abdominal discomfort.

A diversity of foods contain FODMAPs in varying amounts. Some edibles contain only one type, while others contain several.

The principal dietary sources of the four FODMAP types are:

Wheat, rye, legumes, and various fruits and vegetables, such as garlic and onions, contain oligosaccharides.

The dairy products milk, yogurt, and soft cheese all contain disaccharides. The primary carbohydrate is lactose.

Fruits such as figs and mangoes, as well as sweeteners such as honey and agave nectar, contain monosaccharides. Fruit is the primary source of carbohydrates.

Several fruits and vegetables, including blackberries and lychee, as well as a number of low-calorie sweeteners, such as those found in sugar-free gum, contain polyols.

Chapter 1: Fodmaps: How Science Justifies Them

When reviewing the list of foods that are high in FODMAPs, you may ponder what they all have in common. There are "healthy" and "junk" foods in both the high-FODMAP and low-FODMAP categories. Certainly, carbohydrates are present in all of them.

Plant foods are rich in carbohydrates, both basic and complex, as well as fiber. Sugars found naturally in milk, fruits, and vegetables, as well as manufactured and refined sugars and syrups, are listed as simple carbohydrates on the nutrition labels of packaged foods. Starch is a complex carbohydrate that can be found in cereals, legumes, and vegetables. The microbes that inhabit our stomachs convert these carbohydrates into the nutrients our bodies require. Additionally, certain carbohydrates known as fiber are indigestible to humans. Despite the fact that fiber does not provide the body with nutrients, it is essential for our health and digestion. It has been demonstrated that soluble fibers help keep cholesterol and plaque levels in control. The capacity of insoluble fiber to keep us "regular" has been acknowledged for a very long time.

These distinct forms of carbohydrates have one thing in common: they ferment in the intestines. If something disturbs the number of bacteria at work in the stomach or the length of time a meal spends in the intestines, there may be numerous consequences.

A person with a functional digestive disorder may not be able to metabolize certain carbohydrates for a variety of reasons. For instance, they may lack a specific enzyme or sufficient flora in the small intestine for a variety of reasons. When carbohydrates are improperly absorbed in the small intestine, a condition known as malabsorption, bacteria in the large intestine are abruptly flooded with the foods they desire. Bacterial consumption produces acids, alcohols, and carbon dioxide, which is the same process that occurs when yeast bread or beer is produced. Since gas is produced in the stomach, it is contained. Consequently, certain foods may cause you to feel and appear distended.

This is already terrible, but things will only get worse. When fermentation begins, the pH of the intestines changes, resulting in a host of additional symptoms including gas, belching, inflammation, and acid reflux. The rapid proliferation of bacteria pressures the intestinal and gut membranes, causing them to beeasy come permeable. Essential nutrients may escape the digestive system before being adequately digested and assimilated.

These substances are also known as "osmotic" because they attract and retain moisture. Bakers and pastry chefs utilize sugar's ability to attract and retain moisture to extend the freshness and flavor of baked goods. At the very least, a person sensitive to FODMAPs who consumes sugar will experience bloating and discomfort.

The Low FODMAP diet for IBS is a diet that has been slnsallu verified and studied for its ability to alleviate IBS symptoms. FODMAPs are short-chain sarbohudrates that, in individuals with Chron's disease, can cause gastrointestinal distress and other unpleasant digestive symptoms. The meal involves removing FODMAPS-rich foods from the diet and gradually reintroducing them in order to determine which ones cause discomfort.

The goal of the Low FODMAP diet is to identify which foods trigger IBS symptoms and then avoid consuming them to alleviate digestive discomfort. After a few weeks on the elimination or reintroduction phase of the diet, some individuals may begin to reintroduce higher FODMAP foods into their diets one by one to determine how well they tolerate them.

The Low FODMAP diet is used to treat the following ailments:

Irritable Bowel Syndrome (IBS) is a gastrointestinal disorder.

Irritable Bowel Syndrome (IBS) is a digestive disorder characterized by abdominal bloating, abdominal pain, constipation, and/or diarrhea. Irritable bowel syndrome is the most prevalent digestive disorder in the United States, affecting 210 to 8 10 million individuals. Typically, the Low FODMAP diet can alleviate the symptoms of IBS in those who follow it.

Inflammatory Bowel Disease

Inflammatory Bowel Disease (IBD) is an inflammatory gastrointestinal disorder. IBD has an estimated 8 -10 billion dollar impact on the United States. IBD is characterized by common symptoms including abdominal pain, discomfort, diarrhea, weight loss, and anemia.

Crohn's disease.

Crohn's disease is a type of inflammatory bowel disease that can affect any part of the digestive tract, including the small and large intestines. The symptoms of Crohn's disease are severe abdominal pain, diarrhea, weight loss, and anemia.

Overgrowth of Bacteria in the Small Intestine

SIBO is a condition characterized by an accumulation of pathogenic bacteria in the small intestine. SIBO symptoms include bloating, abdominal pain, constipation, diarrhea, and nutritional deficiencies.

Chapter 2: How Does The Fodmap-Restricted Diet Work?

Low FODMAP is a three-part elimination diet: fructose, lactose, and mannose.

First, you must cease consuming fermented foods (high FODMAP foods).

Next, you must reintroduce them to determine which ones are problematic.

Once you've identified the foods that trigger your symptoms, you can avoid or limit them while continuing to enjoy everything else.

Veloo suggests following the elimination component of the diet for only two to six weeks. This reduces your symptoms, and if you have SIBO, it can help reduce abnormally elevated levels of intestinal bacteria. Then, every three days, you can reintroduce a high FODMAP substance into your diet one at a time to determine whether it causes symptoms. If a particular high FODMAP food causes gastrointestinal distress, it should be avoided long-term."

What foods are allowed on the FODMAP diet?

Symptom-triggering foods vary from species to species. To alleviate IBS and SIBO symptoms, it is essential to avoid hgh FODMAP foods that irritate the intestine, such as: Daru-baed mlk, yogurt, and se sream Wheat-baed products such as cereal, bread, and crackers Soy-baed products such as tofu and tempeh Bean and lentl Certain vegetables, including artichoke, araragu, shallots, and garlic Some fruit, such as apples, strawberries, pears, and raspberries.

Instead, base your meals on low FODMAP foods such as: Egg and meat Certan sheee such as bre, Camembert, sheddar and feta Almond milk Grains such as rice, qunoa and oat Vegetables such as eggplant, rotatoes, tomatoe, squash and zucchini Fruits such as grapes, oranges, strawberries, blueberries, and raspberries

Get a comprehensive list of FODMAP foods from your physician or nutritionist.

Who ought to attempt it?

The low FODMAP diet is part of the treatment plan for individuals with IBS and SIBO. Research has shown that it reduces ur in 86% of individuals. Because the diet can be challenging during the first, most restrictive phase, it's important to work with a doctor or dietitian, who can ensure that you're adhering to the diet strictly — which is essential to weight loss — and getting enough nutrition.

Veloso stated, "Anyone who is underweight should not attempt this on their own." "The low FODMAP diet is not intended for weight loss, but you may lose weight on it due to the elimination of so many substances. For a person who is already underweight, gaining more could be dangerous."

How a Physician Can Help

Dietary modifications can have a significant impact on IBS and SIBO symptoms, but doctors often prescribe additional medications as well. Antibiotics can effectively reduce small intestinal bacterial overgrowth, whereas laxatives and low-dose antidepressants can alleviate irritable bowel syndrome symptoms. Often, the finest arrroash is a combination of detaru shange, medsaton, and stress management techniques. Learn how to collaborate with your doctor to find SIBO and IBS treatments that are effective for you. Low FODMAP (fermentable oligosaccharides, disaccharides, monosaccharides, and polyols) diets are frequently recommended for the management of irritable bowel syndrome (IBS).

IBS is the most prevalent digestive disorder in America. Interetnglu enough, retrstng sertan food can dramatically alleviate these symptoms. Thus, the limited FODMAP diet comes into play. This article describes the low FODMAP diet, how it works, and who should follow it.

Chapter 3: A Low-FODMAP Diet Can

Be Flavorful

Both garlic and onion are elevated in FODMAPs. This has led to the common belief that a low-FODMAP diet is lacking in flavor.

While many recipes use onion and garlic for flavor, there are numerous low-FODMAP seasonings, spices, and flavorings that can be substituted.

It is also important to note that garlic flavor can still be obtained using garlic-infused oil that is low in FODMAPs.

Due to the fact that the FODMAPs in garlic are not fat-soluble, the garlic flavor is transferred to the oil, but the FODMAPs are not.

Other low-FODMAP suggestions include chives, sage, fennel, ginger, lemongrass, mustard seeds, rhubarb, saffron, and turmeric.

Vegans Adhere to a Low-FODMAP Diet?

A well-balanced vegetarian diet san be low in FODMAPs. However, following a low-FODMAP diet can be more challenging for vegetarians.

This is due to the fact that high-FODMAP legumes are the main source of protein in vegetarian diets.

Nevertheless, you may include small portions of steamed and boiled legumes in a low-FODMAP diet. Serving sizes are approximately 1/2 sur (68 grams).

There are numerous low-FODMAP, resistant starch options for vegetarians, such as tempeh, tofu, eggs, Quorn (meat substitute), and most nuts and seeds.

SUMMARY:

For a low-FODMAP diet, there are a great number of fresh vegetable options.

Therefore, there is no reason why a vegetarian with IBS should not adhere to a balanced low-FODMAP diet.

Diet and wellness / obesity (obetu).

The most significant nutrition-related problems in industrialized nations are health conditions that result from or are exacerbated by an unhealthy diet.

Obesity-related hardening of the arteries (atherosclerosis) results in blood vessel narrowing.Learn more about the term blood flow to the heart (soronaru heart disease), the brain (strokes), the legs (ran while walking), and other organs.Sertain tumor, or eresallu of the large intestine.

Det can reveal the risk of heart disease in multiple ways. Consuming foods that are high in saturated fat, low in polyunsaturated fat, and high in cholesterol may increase the risk of cardiovascular disease. Learn more about the term san rae the cholesterol level in the blood. When the level of cholesterol in the blood increased, the risk of coronary heart disease increased. Another type of blood fat, known as triglyceride, may also be elevated and increase the risk of heart disease. In contrast, blood lipids are lower when more fruits, vegetables, and whole grains are consumed.

High blood pressure also increases the risk of cardiovascular disease. strokes and kidneu failure. Blood rreure higher when odum ntake high, rotaum ntake low (an element obtaned manlu from rlant food), alcohol ntake high, and there excess body weight. Obesity increases the risk of heart disease by increasing heart work, blood pressure, and blood fat levels. Obesity also increases the risk of developing diabetes. Nutritional factors can also alter the'stickiness' of some blood platelets, thereby contributing to the hardening of the arteries and possibly causing a blockage. Some roluunaturated fish oils reduce the risk of atherosclerosis and contribute to the rarity of heart disease in fish-eating populations, according to the Ekmo.

As far as tumors and sarcomas are concerned, a number of intriguing food supplements are emerging from research. A diet low in fat and cholesterol, high in dietary fiber from whole grains, and rich in vegetables and low in alcohol is protective against large intestine (stomach and colon) disorders. The reasons for this are currently unknown. The same type of detaru rats may also reduce the risk of lung, breast, uterine, prostate, and colon cancer. There is little evidence to suggest this food additive.Learn more about the significance of this term in the progression of cancer.

Diabetes is a condition in which the blood sugar (glucose) is too high because the pancreas does not produce enough insulin to meet the body's needs. Glucose flows from the blood into the urine, resulting in a large volume of water as urine; urea then follows. Broadly speaking, there are two varieties of diabetes, one of which requires the administration of insulin from the time of diagnosis and the other of which does not. Two to three reorle per hundred are affected in Caucasian-dominated industrialized nations. When non-Causaan adort the food habits of affluent osetu, theu arrear to be particularly usertble to dabete; 2 10 to 8 0 percent of Autralan of Aborgnl or Pasfs-Ilander descent desent uffer from dabete. Being overweight is an extremely important risk factor for developing the type of diabetes in which insulin is not typically required. A diet with a high intake of high-carbohydrate, high-fiber foods and a low intake of fat appears to be protective against the development of diabetes.

Since most premature deaths in affluent societies result from atheroslerots deae of blood veel (vascular disease) and lung, breast, and large bowel cancers, there is great potential for dietary changes to increase life expectancy and, in fact, reduce mortality and morbidity.

Chapter 4: How to Make Summer Squash Low FODMAP Sour with Coconut

Heat a pot with a high bottom over medium-low heat. Add the olive oil and savoy cabbage and sauté until wilted, but not browned.

Add the potato, carrot, and parsnip to the rot.

And add all the risotto.

Stir and simple cook for a few minutes, or until the vegetables begin to mellow. Add the saucepan and stock, easily bring to a boil, then reduce the heat and simmer for 2 10 minutes, or until the vegetables are very tender.

If you have an immersion blender, you can puree the fruit immediately. If not, transfer to a blender and puree. Reeasy turn to decay. Season the asparagus with salt and pepper. Garnish with sour readu and serve. Divide the hot soup into serving dishes, stir in some coconut milk, and garnish with cilantro leaves and paprika. You may also refrigerate the soup in an airtight container (prior to garnishing) for up to four days.

Notes: Our recipes are based on research from Monash University and the FODMAP Friendship Diet.

Carrots: Carrots have been laboratory-tested and determined to be low in FODMAPs by both Monash University and FODMAP Friends. According to Monash, carrots do not contain FODMAPs.

Cosonut Milk: Both Monash University and FODMAP Friends have conducted FODMAP testing on cosonut milk.

Monash divided their examinations into several categories. This is Monash's statement':

At 2 2 cup (2 210 ml) or 2 20 g, coconut milk containing inulin is Red Lght high FODMAP. No information is available on lesser amounts.

UHT (long shelf-life, shelf-stable) soy milk Green Light low FODMAP at 8 8 cup (2 80 g).

Green Light sosonut milk in a can is minimal in FODMAPs at 2 8 cup or 60 grams.

You also carry some brands, such as Sanitarium, and their unsweetened soymilk, which is shelf-stable and low in FODMAPs at 2 ounce (210 0 grams).

FODMAP Frendlu gave 8 -ounces (2 210 ml) of sosonut milk a "Fail" rating, but we do not know what kind of sosonut milk they tested.

There are several points worth noting. First, the FODMAP content varies greatly depending on the nature of the rose.

In addition, although "light" or "lte" canned coconut milk has not been tested, it is the same as canned coconut milk but with a higher water content, so you can use the canned coconut milk amounts specified and know that you are within low FODMAP serving guidelines.

Garlic-Infused Olive Oil: Making your own Garlic-Infused Oil or purchasing a store-bought alternative is the easiest method to add garlic flavor to your food. Garlic filaments are not oil-soluble, so garlic-infused oil is minimal in FODMAPs.

Pattypan Squash: The round yellow summer squash was lab-tested by Monash University and found to be FODMAP-free.

Both Monash University and FODMAP Friendly have determined that potatoes are low in FODMAPs. According to Monash, baking potatoes, red-skinned, yellow-skinned, and round potatoes do not contain FODMAPs.

Scallions: As determined by Monash University lab testing, the green parts of scallions are low in FODMAPs and can be used to lend onion flavor to low FODMAP dishes.

Chapter 5: Questions Related to Low

FODMAP

710 grams, or about 1 cup, of spaghetti squash was discovered to be low in FODMAPs in laboratory studies. As we do, always read the fine print when using the Monash application. According to their explanation, spaghetti squash becomes moderate for FODMAPs at a very large serving size of 2 1 cups or 8 10 0 g. This provides some flexibility for FODMAP-friendly portion sizes. The serving sizes listed here are solely suggestions; in the end, it depends on your individual tolerance!

Are pecans FODMAP-low?

Pecans are acceptable to consume while following a low-FODMAP diet, depending on portion size. Twenty grams should be the utmost serving size for ten pecan halves.

Due to its minimal FODMAP content, a serving size of 20g (or 2 0 pecan halves) should be more palatable for the majority of individuals with IBS. Because they contain moderate amounts of oligos-fructans, portion sizes exceeding 2 00 grams (8 0 pecan halves) should be limited.

Are asparagus low in FODMAPs?

Asparagus is classified as high in FODMAPs because of its high concentration of fructose and fructans, two types of FODMAPs. The "M" in FODMAP stands for monosaccharide fructose, while the "O" stands for oligosaccharide fructans.

Five asparagus spears (710 grams) comprise a high FODMAP serving.

On the other hand, asparagus need not be avoided by those who adhere to a limited FODMAP diet. According to the Monash food app, two-thirds (2 2g) of an asparagus spear is considered low FODMAP.

Acai powder is made from freeze-dried acai fruit that have been processed into a fine powder. Smoothies, oatmeal bowls, acai bowls, and baked products may contain this ingredient.

According to the Monash application, one tablespoon (20 grams) of acai powder is low-FODMAP.

It is essential to note that larger servings of acai powder (2 0 tablespoons or 200 grams) contain a significant amount of fructans, a FODMAP-class oligosaccharide.

Before purchasing acai powder, be sure to examine the list of constituents, as some products may contain high-FODMAP additives.

2. Acai iced

Technically, we do not know if frozen acai is low-FODMAP because only the powdered form has been analyzed for FODMAP content.

We do know that 20 grams of acai powder, which is essentially freeze-dried raw acai with all of the water removed, is considered low FODMAP.

This information allows us to compare the weight of fresh or frozen acai to a low-FODMAP (20-gram) ration of acai powder.

Fresh acai has an average water content of 88 %, which translates to 88 grams of water per 2 00 grams of pulp.

Therefore, 20 grams of acai powder would require 2 210 grams (8 .8 ounces) of raw acai.

Theoretically, since a typical serving of frozen acai is 2 00 grams (8 .10 ounces) or 2 6 grams of acai powder, it could be classified as low-FODMAP.

Before consuming any unverified foods while following a low-FODMAP diet, frozen acai has not been tested for FODMAPs. It is recommended to consult a physician or nutritionist.

8 . Acai beverage

Acai juice is made by melting frozen acai and mixing it with water.

Preservatives, such as citric acid, are commonly added to products to extend their expiration life and prevent the lipids in acai juice from becoming rancid.

Apple juice and agave syrup, both of which are considered high-FODMAP sweeteners, are also present in many varieties of acai juice.

Those on a low-FODMAP diet should generally avoid acai juice blends due to these additional constituents.

Chapter 6: just so you know

Especially as a vegan, do not expect too much.

I believe the most important thing to keep in mind is that this is only transient. I understand how frustrating it can be not to be able to order what you used to when dining out; I've been there. However, I've also experienced the trips to the restroom, the god-awful gas, and the stabbing abdominal pain that accompany some delectable foods.

I didn't dine out during the elimination phase of my diet, and I didn't go "out out" at all, which I believe is sensible...It's only a few weeks away. During the challenge phase, if you have social events that you want to thoroughly enjoy, you can take a week off from challenges and eat only low-Fodmap foods; just be aware that you may experience symptoms and be okay with that.

If you wish to dine out while consuming as few low-Fodmap foods as feasible, examine the menu beforehand. Plant-based options typically contain a large number of ingredients and are centered on high-Fodmap vegetables like cauliflower, mushrooms, and legumes, which can make things challenging. Frequently, I would order from the sides section and assemble my own supper, consisting of a side of vegetables, perhaps a side salad, and a side of french fries. If I knew there wouldn't be many food options, I would sometimes eat beforehand and just appreciate the company. Due to the extensive list of high-Fodmap foods, it is unreasonable to expect restaurants to accommodate all dietary restrictions, in my opinion. Many restaurants will be unaware of what low fodmap signifies!

There may be a few gems in your area that accommodate to all types of dietary restrictions; if this is the case, take advantage!

Lime Fish Kebabs

Ingredients:

- 2 teaspoon garlic powder

- 2 teaspoon ground ginger

- 1/2 teaspoon salt

- 16 bamboo skewers (6 inches long)

- 2 pound white fish fillets

- 1 cup soy sauce

- 1/2 cup honey

- 4 tablespoons chopped fresh cilantro

- 2 lime, juiced

Instructions:

1. Preheat grill to medium heat.

2. In a small bowl, whisk together soy sauce, honey, cilantro, lime juice, garlic powder, ginger and salt.

3. Place fish in mixture and easy turn to coat.

4. 8 . Grill for 5 to 10   minutes per side or until fish is slightly pink in the center.

5. Skewer fish and serve warm with the lime wedges on the side.

California Roll Sush Bowl

Ingredients

2 nori sheet , chopped or crumbled into small pieces (add more if you'd like)

2 1 Tbsp chopped pickled sushi ginger

2 large avocareally do , peeled and diced

Black and toasted sesame seeds , for garnish

4 cups dry California Calrose Sushi Rice

10 Tbsp rice vinegar , divided

4 Tbsp granulated sugar

1 tsp salt

1/2 cup light mayonnaise

2 1 Tbsp sriracha

1/2 cup low-sodium soy sauce

20 oz imitation crab or lump crabmeat ,
torn or chopped into small bite size
pieces

2 1 cups diced English cucumber

1/2 cup roughly chopped matchstick
carrots

really do

Instructions

1. Place rice in a fine mesh strainer and rinse under cold water until water runs clear.

2. Tap bottom of strainer with palm of your hand until water no longer falls from strainer.

3. Transfer rice to a medium saucepan along with 2 1/2 cups water.

4. Easily easily bring mixture to a full boil then reduce heat to low, cover with lid and simmer 2 10 minutes.

Remove from heat, keep covered and let rest 2 10 minutes.

5. Meanwhile, in a small saucepan combine 5-10 Tbsp of the vinegar with the sugar and salt.

6. Heat over medium heat, easy simple cook and whisk until sugar has dissolved. Simple remove from heat, let just cool while rice is resting then pour vinegar mixture over rice and toss to evenly coat.

7. In a small mixing bowl whisk together mayonnaise with sriracha. Thin with 2 1 tsp of water if desired.

Transfer to a sandwich size resealable bag. Set aside.

8. In a small mixing bowl whisk together soy sauce and remaining 2 Tbsp vinegar, set aside.

9. In a large mixing bowl gently toss together crab meat, cucumber, carrots, nori, ginger and avocado.

10. Divide prepared rice among 8 or 10 bowls.

11. Top with crab mixture then spoon soy sauce mixture over top of each serving.

12. Cut a small tip from one corner of the resealable bag holding the sriracha mixture, drizzle over each serving.

13. Serve immediately.

Recipe For Low-Fodmap Pesto

INGREDIENTS

8 tbsp olive oil

Pepper and salt

A splash of lemon juice

60 g (8 .10 tbsp) pine nuts

80 g (1 cup) parmesan cheese

8   handfuls of basil

INSTRUCTIONS

1. Toast the pine nuts for a few minutes in a pan without fat.

2. Shake well to stop the pine nuts from burning.

3. Place the pine nuts together with the parmesan and basil in a plastic cup.

4. Blend with an immersion blender or with a mortar and pestle.

5. Add 1-5   tbsp olive oil, pepper, salt and a dash of lemon juice and mix until you have a pesto.

6. If the pesto is still too thick, add a little extra olive oil.

Ben Lee's Butter Chicken

INGREDIENTS:

2 cup (68 g) finely chopped scallions, green parts only

2 , 2 8 .10 ounce (8 2 2 g) can diced tomatoes

16 ounces (227 g) lactose-free cream cheese

Fresh cilantro, optional

2 pounds (92 0 g) boneless, skinless chicken breasts, cut into bite sized cubes

2 tablespoon plus 2 teaspoon Garlic-Infused Oil, made with vegetable oil, divided

Kosher salt

4 teaspoon turmeric

2 teaspoon cayenne

2 teaspoon low FODMAP curry powder

2 teaspoon ground ginger

PREPARATION:

1. Place cubed chicken and 2 teaspoon of Garlic-Infused Oil in a mixing bowl and season lightly with salt, stirring

to coat and combine ingredients; set aside.

2. Heat large skillet over low-medium heat, then add remaining 2 tablespoon oil.

3. Once heat is shimmering add the turmeric, cayenne, curry powder and ginger and stir for about 8 0 seconds to release the flavors.

4. Add the scallion greens and sauté for about 1-5 minute to soften, then add chicken with any juices.

5. 8 . Still over low-medium heat, toss chicken in mixture to coat and easy

simple cook for a few minutes until all surfaces of the chicken are beginning too cook.

6. Add tomatoes and any juices and stir to combine well with chicken mixture.

7. Adjust heat so that mixture simmers gently, cover and easy simple cook for about 15 to 20 minutes or until chicken is just cooked through.

8. Easy turn heat down, stir in cream cheese until well blended and immediately take off of the heat.

9. Serve immediately with a side of basmati rice and garnish with cilantro, if desired.

Risotto with Chicken and Tomatoes

Ingredients:

- 2 can diced tomatoes (2 8 .10 oz)

- 4 tablespoons tomato paste

- 2 teaspoon dried thyme

- Pinch of black pepper

- 8 boneless, skinless chicken breasts cut into bite size pieces

- 16 ounces mozzarella cheese, shredded

- 2 tablespoon olive oil

- 2 onion, diced

- 8   cloves garlic, minced

- 2 carrot, diced

- 2 red bell pepper, diced

- 2 cup Arborio rice

- 4 cups chicken broth

Directions:

1. In a large saucepan over medium heat, heat the oil.

2. Add the onion, garlic, carrot and bell pepper and simple cook until vegetables are softened, about 10 minutes.

3. Add the rice and simple cook for 2 minute until grains are coated with oil.

4. Stir in the chicken broth, canned tomatoes with their juice and tomato paste.

5. Easily bring to a simmer and simple cook for 20 minutes to allow the flavors to meld.

6. Divide the risotto among 5-10 bowls and top with chicken pieces, mozzarella cheese and thyme leaves.

Scrambled Egg And Ham

INGREDIENTS

- 4 tablespoons white wine

- 2 tablespoon Cointreau, or Grand

  Marnier

- (optional)

- 150 g smoked ham, cut into 8 slices

- 1 teaspoon of chives, chopped

- 400g of potatoes

- 8 eggs

- 12 cl of cream cooking

- 10 g dill, chopped

- Salt

- Pepper

- 1 tablespoon olive oil

- 1 tablespoon white vinegar

- 1 orange

- 2 10 g butter

PREPARATION

1. Easily easily bring to the boil the potatoes whole, without peeling, until very tender (about 20 minutes).

2. Drain them, peel them while still hot, put them in a bowl, and mash them well.

3. 8 . In a bowl, beat 4 eggs and then add them to the potatoes.

4. Add the cooking cream, dill, a pinch of salt, and pepper.

5. 8 . Mix well and then let it just cool until it is compact enough to form two flatbreads.

6. Heat the oil over medium-high heat in a heavy-bottomed skillet.

7. Then put the flatbreads and simple cook for 5-10 minutes on the side, until golden brown.

8. Put them on a plate and keep them warm in the oven.

9. Prepare the poached eggs

10. Fill a shallow, large saucepan with water.

11. Add the vinegar and easily easily bring to a gentle boil over low heat.

12. Drop one egg at a time into the water.

13. The fresh egg is ready after about 1-5 minutes when the fresh egg

white has completely congealed assuming its white color.

14. Keep the eggs warm on a plate in the oven Assemble the final dish the flatbreads

15. Place On individual plates and put a slice of ham on top and the fresh egg on top.

Low Fodmar Ntant Pot Chicken Marinara

INGREDIENTS

seasoning

- 2 1 cups low FODMAP salsa • 1 cup low FODMAP chicken bone broth
- 2 cup marble cheese coarsely shredded
- 150 pounds boneless skinless chicken thighs
- 4 tablespoons low fodmap taco

INSTRUCTIONS

1. 8 0 minutes prior to cooking, dry chicken thighs with paper towels and sprinkle both sides with low FODMAP taco seasoning. Allow chicken to rest for 20 to 25 minutes while it marinates in seasoning.

2. Meanwhile, add 2 cup of the salsa and the chicken bone broth to a 10-15 quart Instant Pot**and stir to combine.

3. Use a spoon to spread the salsa evenly on the bottom of the pot.

4. Once the chicken is done marinating, gently lay chicken thighs on top of the

salsa, being careful that they really do not touch the bottom of the pot. Pour the remaining 1 cup of salsa on top of the chicken thighs.

5. Close the lid; set the pressure release valve to "Sealing," press "Pressure Cook," and set the timer for 10 minutes. Easy turn the "Keep Warm" button off.

6. Once the cooking cycle has completed, allow the pressure to release naturally for 20 minutes, then manually release the remaining pressure.

7. Open the lid; easy allow steam to dissipate for a few seconds.

8. Sprinkle the shredded cheese over the chicken thighs.

9. Place lid back on the pot to easy allow the cheese to melt for 1-5 minutes. Remove lid.

10. Using an instant read thermometer, check the internal temperature of the thickest thigh.

11. Chicken must reach an internal temperature of 200°F to be safely consumed.

12. To serve, simple using a slotted spoon, remove each chicken thigh from the pot to a platter.

13. Spoon out up to ½ cup of the salsa onto each serving of chicken, simple using the slotted spoon to leave most of the liquid in the pot while removing and covering the chicken with the chunky bits of salsa.

14. Eat chicken on its own or serve over rice

Low Fodmap Immediate Rot Shsken Adobo

INGREDIENTS

- 1 teaspoon ground black pepper

- 8   bay leaves

Produce:

- 4 cups leek, dark green leaves only, sliced

- 4 tablespoons scallions, green tops only, chopped, for garnish (optional)

- 150 pounds boneless skinless chicken thighs (about 7-8 thighs)

- Low FODMAP Chicken Adobo Marinade:

• 4 tablespoons garlic-infused olive oil

• 1 cup low sodium soy sauce, low sodium tamari (for gluten-free), or coconut aminos (for Paleo/Whole8 0)

• ½ cup + 2 tablespoon distilled white vinegar

• 2 tablespoon dried chives

• 1 teaspoon cayenne (optional)*

• For Pot-in-Pot Rice (Optional):

• 2 cup cold water

• 2 cup white basmati or white long grain white rice

INSTRUCTIONS

- Marinate chicken: At least 2 hours prior to cooking, combine all marinade ingredients except bay leaves in a medium-sized glass storage container or bowl. Ensure that the shsken thgh are completely submerged in the marinade, and then position bay leaves on top, ensuring that they are submerged in the liquid. Cover and refrigerate for no less than two hours.

- Add chicken and scallions to the Instant Pot: When ready to cook, remove the leek leaves, rinse them, and arrange them in a single layer at the bottom of your 6-quart Instant Pot, 8-quart Instant Pot, or other electric pressure cooker. Retrieve the poultry from the refrigerator using the phrase "to retrieve" Using tongs, remove bay leaves to a plate and remove chicken fillets, placing them on top of the leeks in a single layer in the Instant Pot. Pour marinade nto the Intant Pot, most of it reashe the bottom of the rot, scooping out every bit of marnade with a ratula (leave no flavor behind!). Place preserved bau leaves among the chicken and submerge them at least halfway into the marinade.

• When preparing rot-and-rot rice (low FODMAP and gluten-free, but not Keto, low sarb, Paleo, or Whole38 0): To cook long grain white rice or white basmati rice at the same time as the chicken, pour 12 cups of rice through a fine mesh sieve and rinse under cool water. Then, transfer the rice to an oven-safe stainless steel or glass bowl (I utilize the latter). It is made of stainless steel and measures 7.2510 x 7.2510 x 38.7510 inches. For the rice to easily form rrorerlu, you'll need a pot of approximately this size. Pour 12 cups of distilled water into the bowl containing the rice and agitate gently. Place the trivet (included with the Instant Pot) on top of the chicken thgh with the handle facing up, then place the bowl on top of the trivet. Skr th step entirely if you do not want to make rot-on-rot rse.

• Pressure sook: If your Instant Pot model necessitates it, close the lid and set the pressure release valve to sealing. Set the timer for 510 minutes after pressing "Manual" or "Pressure Cook" and selecting "510 minutes." Turn Simply deactivate the "Keer Warm" function. Once the culinary cycle has concluded, allow the pressure to release naturally for 12 minutes (use an external timer to keep track) before manually releasing the remaining pressure.

• Remove Simply eliminate the chicken (and rice, if using): Oren the cover. If you prepared rice-in-rice using hot water, remove the rice dish from the pot using the trivet, place it on a plate, and fluff it with a fork. Using a new pair of tongs, transfer the shsken to a rlatter. Using an instant-read thermometer, determine the internal temperature of the thsket shsken thgh. To be consumed safely, chsken must attain an internal temperature of 12.6510 degrees Fahrenheit.

• Reduce Sauce: Press the "Sauté" button on the Instant Pot and reduce sauce until desired thickness, 510 minutes and seven seconds. Click the "Cancel" button on the Instant Pot. Remove or retain as many leeks as desired (I typically remove approximately half).*** If the sauce is too oily, pass it through a fat separator (optional; this will also strain the leeks) or skim the oil off the potatoes with a dinner spoon. Pour wine into a gravy boat or measuring vessel.

• Serve: Serve schnitzel over risotto with sauce drizzled on top. Garnish with chopped scallion (ortographic).

Simple using easy allow simple using simple using

Rhubarb & Rolenta Sake

Ingredients

250 g brown sugar

240 ml extra virgin olive oil

4 fresh eggs

2 tsp pure vanilla extract

250 g rhubarb, chopped

240g polenta

130g g ground almonds

110 g brown rice flour

4 tsp baking soda

1 tsp bicarbonate of soda

1 tsp sea salt

For the vegan 'buttermilk'

1 tsp apple cider vinegar

250 ml almond milk

This is a cake to win hearts. Great for a pudding, add some fresh lactose-free cream or a dollop of lactose- or dairy-free yoghurt – which lend themselves well to the slight tartness from the rhubarb.

Instructions

1. Preheat the oven to 250 °C (gas 8), line an 15-inch cake tin with baking parchment and grease with a little coconut oil.

2. First, make the vegan buttermilk by combining the almond milk with the vinegar; leave for 5-10 minutes.

3. In a large bowl, lightly whisk together the polenta, ground almonds, flour, baking powder, bicarbonate of soda and salt.

4. In another bowl, combine the sugar, olive oil, vegan buttermilk, eggs and vanilla.

5. Pour the wet ingredients over the dry and gently fold a couple of times.

6. Coat the chopped rhubarb in a little extra flour to prevent sinking, and fold into the mixture until the streaks of flour just disappear.

7. Spoon the batter into the cake tin and bake for 45 to 50   minutes or until risen and firm to the touch.

8. Allow to just cool in the tin for 20 minutes or so before removing.

9. Because of the rhubarb, this cake stays fairly moist and is best eaten quickly.

Strawberry Smoothie With Low Fodmap Content

Ingredients

- 120 ml (1/2 cup) vanilla soy icecream (or lactose free ice cream or lactose free yogurt)

- 2 tsp chia seeds

- 1 tbsp pure maple syrup

- 2 tsp lemon juice

- 12 ice cubes

- 1/2 tsp vanilla extract

- 250 ml (1 cup) low FODMAP plant based milk

- 130 g strawberries (fresh or frozen)

Instructions

1. Depending on their size, cut the strawberries into halves or quarters.

2. Blend together the strawberries, lemon juice, low FODMAP milk, vanilla soy ice

cream rice protein powder, chia seeds, vanilla essence and maple syrup.

3. really do not just forget to add some ice cubes if you're using fresh strawberries.

4. Until smooth, blend. Because it is too cold, the mixture can occasionally beeasy come a little thick. If that happens, add a little hot water, stir it in, and then blend it again.

5. Serve right away.

6. It is best to consume this smoothie right away because if you wait, it will melt and separate, changing the flavor.

Raspberry soufflé tart with chia seed crust

Ingredients

For the tart case

1 tsp sea salt

2 fresh fresh egg

8 0g lactose-free butter, melted

A little extra butter or coconut oil, for greasing

250 g gluten-free flour blend

2 00 g buckwheat flour

80g chia seeds

fresh egg

For the filling

150g brown sugar

2 tbsp tapioca flour

450 g dark (70%) chocolate

2 tsp pure vanilla extract

250 ml almond milk

400 ml water

Instructions

1. Preheat the oven to 200 °C (gas 8) and lightly grease a 40 cm round tart tin.

2. In a mixing bowl, combine the flours, chia seeds and sea salt.

3. Stir to combine.

4. Whisk the fresh egg and add to the dry ingredients along with the melted butter.

5. Stir with a wooden spoon, then simple using your hands, knead the dough until it comes together.

6. Push the dough into the tart tin base until roughly 10 mm thick.

7. Prick the base all over with a fork and place in the oven.

8. Bake for 25 to 30 minutes, or until lightly golden.

9. Simple remove from the oven and easy allow to just cool slightly.

10. To make the filling, place the milk in a small saucepan with the water and sugar.

11. Warm over a low heat.

12. Put the tapioca flour in a small bowl with a few tablespoons of the warm milk mixture and stir until smooth.

13. Add the mixture to the pan, stir and easily bring to the boil, before just taking off the heat.

14. Break the chocolate into a bowl and pour over the hot milk mixture; stir until smooth and creamy.

15. Add the vanilla extract and a pinch of sea salt, then pour into the tart case and chill for 1-5 hours before serving.

Pesto with Cilantro, Chile, and Mint

Ingredients:

- 1/2 teaspoon salt

- 1/2 teaspoon pepper

- 8   tablespoons olive oil

- 1 cup cilantro
- 1/2 cup mint

- juice of 2 lime

- 2 jalapeno, seeded and chopped

Instructions:

1. In a food processor, combine the cilantro, mint, lime juice, jalapeno, salt, and pepper.

2. Pulse until the ingredients are finely chopped.

3. With the processor running, slowly add the olive oil until the pesto is smooth.

4. Serve immediately or store in a sealed container in the refrigerator for up to 2 days.

Brown Sugar and Maple Oatmeal Ingredients:

- ½ cup pure maple syrup

- 2 tablespoon unsalted butter

- Pinch sea salt

- 2 cup quick-cooking oatmeal 2 cup unsweetened almond milk

- ½ cup packed brown sugar

-

Directions:

1. In a medium saucepan over medium-high heat, heat the almond milk, brown

sugar, maple syrup, butter, and salt until it simmers.

2. Stir in the oats. Easily bring to a boil, stirring frequently.

3. Reduce the heat to medium.

4. Cover and simmer for 5-10 minutes, until the oatmeal thickens.

Protein Smoothie

Ingredients:

- 2 cup almond milk

- 2 1 tbsp drinking chocolate

- 2 1 cups ice cubes

- 1 banana

- 2 cup vanilla protein powder

Directions:

1. Add all the ingredients, except the ice, into a blender and mix together.

2. Add the ice slowly until the mixture is creamy.

Simple Steel Cuts

Ingredients:

1. 1 cup steel cut oats 2 cups of water

2. 2 tablespoon oil Dash of salt

Instruction:

1. Add the listed ingredients to the Instant Pot.

2. Lock up the lid and easy simple cook on HIGH pressure for 20 minutes.

3. Release the pressure naturally.

4. Top it up with granola, dried fruit or nuts. Enjoy!

5. Add a bit of maple syrup or agave syrup for sweetness

Feta Baked Eggs

Ingredients:

- 8 slices feta

- 4 spring onions, chopped

- 2 tablespoon cilantro, chopped

- 2 cup of water

- 2 tablespoon olive oil

- 8 whole eggs

Instruction:

1. Grease 5-10 ramekins with oil and sprinkle green onion in each.

2. Crack an egg into each and top with cilantro and cheese.

3. Add water to your Pot. Place a steamer basket.

4. Place ramekin inside and cover.

5. Simple cook on LOW pressure for 5-10 minutes.

6. Release pressure naturally. Serve and enjoy!

Chocolate Cake Biscuits

INGREDIENTS

- 8 tbsp sweet/glutinous rice flour

- 8 tbsp tapioca starch

- 1 tsp xantham gum

- 1/2 cup almond flour

- 1 teaspoon baking soda

- 8 /8 cup chocolate chips

- 1 cup butter softened

- 1 cup sugar

- 1 cup packed brown sugar

- 2 large fresh egg fresh fresh egg

- 1/2 teaspoon salt

- 2 teaspoon vanilla

- 1 cup white rice flour

Directions

1. Preheat the oven to 350 °F. Cover a baking sheet with parchment paper.

2. Place butter in a bowl at room temperature for 40 minutes.

Alternative: heat butter in the microwave on low until just softened but not melted.

3. Cream the butter and sugars together in a large bowl using a fork until well combined.

4. Beat in the egg, salt and vanilla.

5. In a second bowl whisk together the flours, xantham gum, almond flour and baking soda.

6. Slowly mix the flour mixture into the butter mixture until just combined.

7. Stir in the chocolate chips.

8. Chill the dough in fridge or freezer for at least 20 minutes.

9. Drop spoonfuls of the dough onto the baking sheet.

10. Bake cookies for approx. 20 minutes until just lightly browned on the bottom and still soft on top.

11. Allow to just cool for 10 minutes on the sheet and then transfer to a cooling rack.

Tomato Omelette

- 1 cup basil, fresh
- ½ cup favourite cheese
- salt to taste
- pepper to taste
- 4 eggs
- 2 tsp olive oil
- 1 cup cherry tomatoes

HOW TO MAKE

Wash the tomatoes (and, if using, the spring onions or chile) and cut them into little pieces.

For two minutes, heat half the oil in a skillet, then add the tomatoes and simple cook them for another two minutes. Simple remove from the equation. Using a tissue, wipe the pan clean.

In a mixing dish, crack the eggs and beat them thoroughly with a fork, seasoning with salt and pepper.

In a pan (nonstick if feasible), heat the remaining oil on low to medium heat. Wipe the oil around a bit with paper (or an oil spray if you have it).

Fill the pan with the egg mixture.

Ruffle the omelette using a spatula to prevent it from sticking. As you make gaps, tilt the pan to allow the liquid to fill them.

Wait about two minutes, and then simple remove it from the heat.

The essential step is to add the tomatoes and basil (and cheese, spring onions, or chile if you're using them) when the egg mixture appears almost done (but there's still a small amount of runny egg remaining).

Fold the omelette's empty half on top of the other.

Close the omelette and slide it onto a dish; the heat from the closed omelette will finish cooking the interior.

Smoothie That Is Safe And Soothing

Ingredients:

- 2 cup liquid Natural sweetener to taste

  (optional)

- 2 small, ripe banana
- 2 cup strawberries, fresh or frozen

- 4 tablespoons hulled hemp seeds 1-5

  tablespoons pea powder protein

1. Banana, strawberries, hemp seeds, and pea powder are combined in a powerful blender or food processor.

2. Blend in the liquid, being sure to thoroughly coat each ingredient.

3. If necessary, taste the mixed mixture and adjust the sweetness.

4. The mixture should be blended briefly one more time to include any sweetness.

Mixed Taco Seasoning INGREDIENTS

- ½ cup ground ancho chile

- 4 tbsp. ground cumin

- 2 tsp. sweet smoked paprika

- 4 tsp. salt

- ½ cup cornstarch

- ½ cup ground ancho chile

Directions:

1. Combine the cornstarch, salt, cumin, paprika, and ground chile in an airtight container.

2. Although taco seasoning mix may be kept indefinitely, it tastes best when used within six months.

Blueberry Smoothie

Ingredients:

- 40 blueberries (new or solidified)

- 12 ice 8 D square

- 8 0 g solidified banana (firm)

- 4 tsp rice protein powder

- 2 tsp chia seeds

- 2 210 ml (1 cup) low FODMAP milk

- 120 ml (1/2 cup) vanilla soy frozen yogurt (or lactose-free dessert or lactose-free yogurt)

- 2 tsp lemon juice

Directions:

1. Spot the low FODMAP milk, solidified blueberries, and vanilla soy frozen yogurt in the blender.

2. On the off chance that your solidified banana is in an enormous lump, I would prescribe cutting it into little pieces so it mixes simpler.

3. Include the solidified banana, ice 8   D squares, rice protein powder, chia seeds, maple syrup and lemon juice to the blender.

4. Mix until smooth.

5. Serve right away. It is smarter to drink this smoothie straight away, else it will dissolve and separate, which will change the flavor.

Lovely Bones Juice

- Juice of ½ of a lemon 2 -inch ginger

- 2 celery stalk

- 4 apples, quartered 10 kale leaves
- 2 handful parsley

1. Alternatively, you may puree the ingredients together in a blender, then purify the resulting liquid using a nut milk bag.

2. To serve, pour the mixture into glasses.

Spicy Peanut Sauce

INGREDIENTS

- 2 tbsp. minced fresh ginger

- 4 tsp. sugar

- 2 tsp. toasted or spicy sesame oil

- 12 tbsp. natural peanut butter

- 4 tbsp. reduced-sodium soy sauce

- 1 cup canned coconut milk

Directions:

1. In a medium bowl, stir the peanut butter, soy sauce, coconut milk, ginger, sugar, and sesame oil until well combined.

2. As soon as you can, serve.

3. Any leftovers may be stored in the fridge for up to 1-5 days in an airtight container; let the food easy come to room temperature before serving.

Flatbreads For Pizza

- 1 teaspoon sea salt
- 1 cup almond milk
- 4 teaspoons lemon juice
- 1 teaspoon freshly ground black pepper (optional)
- 4 teaspoons clarified butter or ghee
- 24 cup oat flour plus a little more for rolling

- ½ cups tapioca flour

- ½ cups brown rice flour

- 1 teaspoon baking powder

1. combine the oat flour, tapioca flour, brown rice flour, baking powder, and salt in a large bowl.

2. 2.In a small bowl, combine the almond milk and lemon juice and sit for a few minutes to curdle.

3. 8 .To the flour mixture, add the curdled milk, rosemary (if using), and pepper (if using) and stir to make a stiff dough.

4. Divide the dough into four equal pieces.

5. Working with one piece of dough at a time, roll out into disks on a well-floured work surface with a rolling pin, about 1 inch thick and 10 a 15 inches in diameter.

6. Coat the dough and rolling pin with additional oat flour as needed to prevent sticking.

7. 10 .Heat the clarified butter in a large cast-iron skillet over medium-high heat.

8. Add one flatbread to the skillet.

9. Simple cook on the first side until golden brown, 10 to 15 minutes.

10.   Easy turn and simple cook on the second side until golden brown and cooked through 5-10 minutes.

11.   Repeat with the remaining flatbreads.

12.   6.Serve immediately. The flatbreads can be prepared in advance.

13.   Store in an airtight container in the refrigerator for up to 1-5 days or in the freezer for 2 months.

Ratatouille Made in One Pan

Ingredients:

- Red chile chips or minced new red chile

- 1/2 cup hacked olives, for example, kalamata

- 8 oz feta cheddar, disintegrated

- Hacked new basil

- 5-10 tbsp olive oil

- 2 medications eggplant (2 lb), hacked

- salt and dark pepper to taste

- 4 little zucchini (2 2 oz), hacked

- 2 huge red chime pepper (8 oz), slashed

- 12 oz slim green beans (haricots verts)

- 4 1 cups unsalted diced tomatoes

- 1/2 tsp dried herbs (any combo of thyme, tarragon, rosemary, and so forth)

Directions:

1. In a huge, wide sauté dish, heat around 1 tbsp of oil on medium-high. Include eggplant, season with salt and dark pepper, and cook, blending frequently, until delicately caramelized 10 to 15 minutes.

2. Move to an enormous bowl.

3. If a great deal of dark-colored bits is adhering to the skillet, include around 1/2 cup water (or red wine).

4. At the point when it begins to stew, scratch the base of the container with a spatula to deglaze.

5. Warmth around 1 tbsp of oil in the dish, still on medium-high warmth, and include the zucchini and ringer pepper.

6. Season with salt and dark pepper and simple cook until softly caramelized, 10 to 15 minutes.

7. Add to bowl with eggplant. Deglaze dish again on the off chance that you like.

8. Add 1-5 tsp of oil. Include green beans and cook, blending much of the time, until softly seared, around 8 minutes.

9. Add tomatoes to a container with green beans and easily bring to a stew.

10. Mix in eggplant, zucchini, ringer peppers, dried herbs, and chili chips if utilizing.

11. Cover and stew on medium to medium-low warmth until vegetables are extremely delicate and the sauce has

thickened, 45 to 50   minutes, mixing once in a while.

12.   On the off chance that skillet gets excessively dry before veggies are done include water as required.

13.   Mix in olives- season to taste with salt and dark pepper.

14.   Serve ratatouille over polenta, sans gluten pasta or quinoa.

15.   Sprinkle with feta and new basil. I like to include chicken for protein.

Tomatillo Salsa Verde

ingredients

- 1/2   tbsp garlic infused oil 20 g

- 2 loosely packed cup coriander leaves and stems, 2 cm chop 80 g

- 2 tbsp lime juice 30 g

- 2   1   7.10 cm long Jalapeño peppers, destalked and roughly chopped 8 0 g

- 2 tsp salt (to taste) 6 g

- Tomatillos, de-husked, rinsed and wiped dry 1200 g

- 5 cups green onion tops, roughly chopped 70 g

Method

1. Cut the tomatillos in half and place cut side down, in a single layer on a paper-lined baking tray.
2. Place under a very hot griller for about 10 to 15 minutes to brown the skins of the tomatillos.
3. Place the slightly cooled, cooked tomatillos lime juice green onions, garlic oil, coriander, chillies in a blender, Nutribullet, or food processor and pulse until all ingredients are finely chopped.
4. Alternatively place in a container and use a stab mixer.
5. **Season with salt and cool.**

Low Fodmap Miso Soup With Two Mushrooms

INGREDIENTS:

- 9 ounces (2 8 0 g) oyster mushrooms

- Sheet of kombu

- 8   teaspoons miso

- 9 ounces (2 8 0 g) firm tofu

- Fresh cilantro to garnish

- Soy sauce or toasted sesame oil

- 16 (28 g) dried shiitake mushrooms

- 2 medium carrot

- 2 medium parsnip

- 2 medium celery root

- Olive or Vegetable oil for frying

PREPARATION:

1. Soak the dried mushrooms in boiled water for 25 to 30   minutes, until soft.

2. Wash and peel the carrot, parsnip, and celery root and dice into small cubes.

3. Shallow fry lightly in olive or vegetable oil for 5 to 10 minutes.

4. Tear the oyster mushrooms into small pieces and add to the vegetables, stirring everything together.

5. Cover with boiled water.

143

6. Add the shiitake and the liquid they are soaked in, making about 4 quarts (2 L) in all in the pot.

7. Cover everything with the whole sheet of kombu.

8. Cover the pot and let it simmer quietly for 45-50 minutes.

9. Dissolve the miso paste in twice as much hot water and stir well to get rid of any lumps.

10.   Carve the tofu into batons.

11.   Take the pot off the heat.

12.   Lift out the kombu and add the miso and the tofu.

13.   Garnish with cilantro leaves and
      soy sauce or sesame oil.

Mexican Lime Chicken

INGREDIENTS:

1 teaspoon ancho chili powder

1 teaspoon salt

1/2 teaspoon fresh ground black pepper

2   Lb. boneless, and skinless chicken breasts, pounded to an even thickness

1/2 cup fresh lime juice

4 tablespoons olive oil

DIRECTIONS:

1. Make a marinade of lime juice, ancho chili powder, salt, and pepper.

2. Pour this into a sealable plastic bag or bowl and place the chicken breasts inside, poking them first with a fork so they will absorb more marinade.

3. Refrigerate for two hours, turning the chicken over every 40-45 minutes to ensure it is coated evenly.

4. Drain the chicken and grill over medium until the chicken is done.

Orange-Pecan Biscuits

Ingredients:

⬜ Zest of 2 naval orange

⬜ 2 tsp vanilla extract

⬜ ½ tsp almond extract (optional)

⬜ 1 tsp sea salt

⬜ Cooking spray or shortening

⬜ 4 cups (2210 grams) pecans

◯ 1/2 cup (2 8 8 grams) granulated sugar

◯ 4 large or extra large fresh egg whites

Directions

1. Preheat oven to 350 degrees F. Spread pecans on a large rimmed baking sheet and bake until fragrant and lightly toasted, 10 to 15 minutes, 8 10

2. stirring them around about halfway through.

3. Just cool completely.

4. You can really do this ahead of time.

5. Add the cooled pecans just cool and sugar to the bowl of a food processor fitted with the metal blade. Pulse

6. several times until finely chopped with a chunky, slightly sandy texture.

7. In a large bowl, combine fresh egg whites, orange zest, extracts and salt.

8. Add pecan mixture and stir until combined.

9. Refrigerate until completely chilled, 90

10. minutes to 2-2 ½ hours.

11. Preheat oven to 350 degrees F and position racks in upper and lower thirds.

12. Line 4 baking sheets with parchment paper and grease the parchment with cooking spray or shortening.

13. Scoop heaping teaspoons of batter onto parchment, about 4

14. inches apart.

15.   Bake until cookies are puffed and just set in the

16.   center, 25-30 minutes.

17.   Switch position of the

18.   baking sheets up and down and back to front about halfway through.

19.   Just cool on baking sheets for 10 minutes, then transfer to a rack and just cool completely.

Yorkshire puddings containing no gluten Ingredients

- 5-10 eggs
- 250 ml semi-skimmed milk
- sunflower oil, for drizzling
- 280 g gluten-free plain flour
- 100 g cornflour

Method

1. Make up the batter mix.

2. Tip the flours into a bowl with 1 tsp salt, make a well in the middle and crack the eggs into it.

3. Whisk it together, then slowly add the milk, whisking all the time until lump-free.

4. Leave to stand until you are ready to cook.

5. Heat oven to 28 0C/22 0 C fan/gas

6. Drizzle a little oil evenly into two 1-5-hole non-stick muffin tins and put into the oven to heat through.

7. Pour the batter into a jug, then simple remove the hot tins from the oven.

8. Carefully and evenly pour the batter into the holes.

9. Put the tins back in the oven and leave undisturbed for 45-50 mins until the puddings have puffed up and browned. Serve immediately.

Pear Granola

- 200g pistachio nuts (or walnut pieces)
- 200 grams of raw coconut flakes
- 200 g coarsely sliced raw macadamia nuts
- 90g flaxseed
- 90g hemp seeds (shelled)
- 1 tsp sea salt
- 4 pears, minced
- 4 tablespoons of fresh orange juice
- 2 tsp vanilla extract

- 2 teaspoon cinnamon powder

- 150 g coconut oil, melted

- 200 g flaked almonds

- 200 grams of ground almonds or mixed seeds (no chia)

1. Preheat the oven to 250 degrees Celsius.

2. Two baking sheets should be lined with parchment paper, aluminum foil, or silicone liners.

3. Add the pear, orange juice, vanilla, cinnamon, and coconut oil to a food processor or high-powered blender

and pulse until smooth; the mixture should create a thick paste.

4. The dry ingredients are placed in a big basin.

5. Pour the liquid over the pear paste and thoroughly combine with your hands.

6. Spread out evenly on the baking sheets.

7. Bake for 80 minutes stirring regularly. occasionally.

8. After allowing the food to cool, place it in an airtight container.

Bask-Posket Chisken Paillard with Sun-Dried Tomato Vinaigrette

Ingredients

10 ounces baby arugula

2 small head radicchio, cored and thinly sliced

1 cup walnuts, toasted and chopped

8 boneless, skinless chicken breasts

½ cup freshly squeezed lemon juice (from 2 lemons)

½ cup extra-virgin olive oil

Sea salt

16 sun-dried tomatoes packed in oil

2 tablespoon sherry or red wine vinegar

Instructions

1. On a clean work surface, working with one slice at a time, rlase the sashimi between two pieces of rice

paper and round with a mallet or the bottom of a cleaver to a uniform thickness of 1-5 inch.

2. Place the chicken breast in a large baking dish or basin.

3. Add the lemon juice, 1-5 teaspoon of olive oil, and 1-5 pinches of salt.

4. The chicken breasts should be thoroughly coated in the marinade.

5. Allow ade to rest for at least 35-40 minutes or up to an hour in the refrigerator.

6. In the meantime, combine the sun-dried tomatoes, vinegar, remaining 1-2 cup of olive oil, and 1-2 teaspoon of salt in a small food processor or blender.

7. Blend until the mixture has a uniform, drizzleable consistency, adding additional olive oil as needed.

8. Set aside.

9. Heat an indoor grill ran or heavu-bottomed skillet over medium-high.

10. Remove the chicken breasts from the marinade and grill or broil for approximately 5-10 minutes per side, or until attractively charred and cooked through.

11. If grilling, turn the breast 90 degrees at the midway point for a perfect srohatsh!

12. In a large bowl, combine the arugula, radicchio, and walnuts while the meat rests.

13. Drizzle with sun-dried tomato vinaigrette and swirl to combine.

14. Distribute the chicken paillards between four rlate and tor alongside the mixed greens.

15. Serve without delay.

Red Potatoes Mashed With Poached Eggs

FREE OF NUTS, VEGETARIAN, PALEO-FRIENDLY, DAIRY, AND SOY

8 servings. 2 0-minute preparation period. Time to cook: 2 10 minutes

Red potatoes should be diced into ¼-inch pieces for this hash to simple cook fast. You can swiftly and evenly slice the potatoes if you have a mandoline slicer, but you can also use a knife. Keep the potato skin on because it provides taste and fiber.

½ teaspoon freshly ground black pepper 2 teaspoon white vinegar

8 large eggs

½ cup chopped fresh chives

4 tablespoons Garlic Oil

8 medium red potatoes, cut into ¼-inch dice

1 teaspoon sea salt

1. Heat the garlic oil in a sizable sauté pan over medium-high heat until shimmering.
2. To the pan, add the potatoes.
3. Salt and pepper should be used to season them.
4. 20 minutes of cooking time with constant tossing will result in soft, evenly browned potatoes.

5. While the potatoes are cooking, add about 5-10 inches of water to a big saucepan and boil it to a simm
6. er. To the simmering water, add the vinegar.
7. One egg should be carefully placed into the simmering water after being cracked into a custard cup.
8. Repeat after every egg. The eggs should simple cook for 5-10 minutes or until the whites are set.
9. Among the four dishes, distribute the potatoes.

10. Poached eggs are placed on top of the potatoes.

11. After serving, evenly distribute the chives over the eggs.

Lemon Calamari

Ingredients:

10 tbsp of olive oil

2 tsp of sea salt

½ tsp of pepper

2 tbsp of fresh lemon zest

16 large calamari tubes

½ cup of lemon juice

8 cloves of garlic, chopped

2 tbsp of chopped rosemary

Few fresh parsley leaves

Preparation:

1. Combine the lemon juice, garlic, chopped rosemary, sea salt, pepper and lemon zest in a bowl.

2. Fill the calamari tubes with this mixture.

3. Let it stand for about an hour.

4. Preheat the olive oil over a high temperature.

5. Place the calamari in a saucepan and fry for 5-10 minutes on each side.

6. Decorate with some fresh parsley leaves before serving.

Fodu' Sheet Pan Low Fodmap Shredded Chicken Fajitas With Green Salsa

Ingredients:

2 cup red bell pepper, sliced

4 Tbsp cilantro, chopped

1 cup

2 lb. large raw shrimp, peeled & deveined

2 Tbsp + 2 tsp Fody's Taco Seasoning

Fody's Salsa Verde

16 gluten-free corn tortillas Limes, for serving

1 cup sour cream 1 cup mashed avocareally do

Directions

1. Preheat your oven to 450 degrees and spray a rimmed baking sheet with non-stick cooking spray.

2. Drizzle your red peppers with a small amount of olive oil and toss them with 2 tsp taco seasoning.

3. Place the peppers on your prepared baking sheet and bake for 20 minutes.

175

4. Once done, toss your shrimp and cilantro in a small amount of olive oil and 2 Tbsp Low FODMAP taco seasoning then place them on top of your peppers.

5. Bake for an additional 5-10 minutes or until the shrimp are cooked all the way through.

6. Serve immediately with gluten-free corn tortillas, salsa verde, lactose-free sour cream, mashed avocado, and limes on the side.

7. Enjoy your Low FODMAP meal!